```
I0414891
```

Before the Journey

Let me introduce you to the reasons I started this journey. There are some people in my life who mean the world to me. They are at the heart of this amazing journey.

Without the support and understanding of my wife, Amanda, it would be difficult to even be able to do what I have done in the last couple of years. She has stuck by my side through thick and thin. When times were tough she remained the one constant outside my relationship with God. Having a strong marriage is important. Many times, when trouble arises, and things become difficult a spouse may flee the marriage. This wasn't the case with Amanda.

Preface

This story is about a journey which started 13 years ago. I learned what it means to be committed to a process, regardless of what that process involves. I learned about the importance of living a healthy lifestyle and how your health can affect everything in your life. Everything from family to financial wellbeing. I learned about the importance of keeping God first in your life and how he will guide you through any situation regardless how hard. Join me as I share my story of faith & witness, a journey to a new me.

Index

The other people in my life who have been important to me on this journey are my girls, Bethany and Bailey. You will learn more about Bethany, but she taught me what it means to be a fighter. Then there's Bailey, the little girl who shows those puppy dog eyes to daddy to get her way.

My parents have been an amazing support. I have always looked up to my dad from the time I was a child. I truly believe he was the example for me to follow and look up to. I want to be that same kind of example for my girls.

My mother is very proud of me for being able to have my life and health restored. She prays for me daily. We talk every morning between 6:00 and 7:00 on my way to work.

There will be others to meet along this journey. It is my prayer that as you follow me on this journey you experience God's best. So, sit back and enjoy as I take you on a journey that started in April 2017 it truly started in August 2006.

The Journey Begins

2006 was a hard year for Amanda and me. I lived several years blind to the possibility that my weight could contribute to health problems as I got older. My dad was diagnosed with Type 2 diabetes when I was a freshman in college and there was a history of diabetes in my family. Even though the family history was there I never saw myself in this position. I never saw myself being diagnosed with diabetes. Little did I know my life was about to change. Not only my life, but mine and Amanda's marriage.

The exact date is a blur but what I do remember is how what happened became seared in my mind. August 2006 the unthinkable happened. I had a pulmonary embolism and was diagnosed with type 2 diabetes. Four months later our oldest daughter, Bethany was born.

Nine weeks premature, tipping the scales at 1 pound 6.5 ounces at birth. She spent the first 4 months of her life in the NICU. She was and still is our miracle from God. She will always be my little lady.

Despite the difficulties we faced, I never really took my health and wellness seriously. I didn't really change my habits. I tried the South Beach diet and I had a gym membership. The struggle to see results wore on me and led to discouragement. Because of the discouragement and frustrations, I gave up. I honestly felt like I was a lost cause.

In 2009, we added to the family with the birth of our youngest daughter, Bailey. Even with two beautiful daughters, I still did not take my health and wellness seriously. It was a struggle for me to get on the floor and play with my girls. I couldn't go outside and play with them without getting winded. My knees would hurt, making it difficult to walk. The girls would want to walk around the neighborhood or ride their bikes, but I didn't because my knees and back would start to hurt.

I wasn't the father my girls needed or deserved. I wanted to be out there walking and playing with them, but deep down inside I became discouraged because I knew how much I would hurt. I was failing as a husband and a father. Amanda and the girls deserved better than what I was giving them. Amanda needed her husband back and the girls needed a daddy they could rely on.

Through everything I had gone through in 2006, my faith in God was tested. I learned a lot about my own personal experiences through the birth of our first child. I learned how much God is in control and how His hands were on my family. But I still struggled to let God have full control of my health and wellness. Because of my unwillingness to let God have control I continued to struggle with my weight.

Those struggles led to several hospitals stays with cellulitis in my legs. Even with that, I kept trying to do it on my own and continued to fail. I wasn't changing what needed to change. I wasn't letting go and letting God.

Finding My Purpose

Almost 2 years ago we started attending Midtowne Church in Benton, Arkansas. We were in a chapter of our life, as a family, where we were between churches and looking for a church home where we were all happy. I received confirmation that Midtowne was our new church home when the pastor preached on pursuing your passions to fulfill God's purpose. For me, what I thought was my passion turned out to just be a hobby.

For the longest, I thought my passion for BBQ was how God would use me to make a difference in the lives of other people. There's nothing like the smell of hickory burning in a smoker. I kept thinking God was going to use BBQ and my enjoyment to make a difference in the lives of other people by feeding the needy. Was I wrong!

God began to speak to me and reveal something about a previous experience never really gave much thought about. When I had my pulmonary embolism, I experienced something which, at the time, I didn't understand. It may be hard for some to comprehend. Even I had a hard time comprehending exactly what had happened.

I had what many would call an out of body experience. For so long, I was scared to talk about it, because I didn't know what others would think. I thought people would look at me like I had was off my rocker.

God began to impress on my heart the need to share that day with other people. He opened the door and gave me the opportunity to share my story with someone at work. Through this opportunity it began to be clear that what I experienced, with the pulmonary embolism, was more than just an out of body experience. God began to reveal a greater meaning.

The moment I passed out, my spirit left my body. It was as if I could look down over the car and see my body lying in the driver's seat. The one thing I remember most is the experience was peaceful.

When you read in the Bible descriptions of hell and how it is a place of torment and darkness, what I experienced was nothing like that. 2 Peter 2:3, "for if God did not spare angels when they sinned, but sent them to hell, putting them in chains of darkness to be held for judgment." I experienced a peaceful reminder that God was in control and had his hands on my life. And when it was time for me to come home, I would indeed spend eternity with Him in heaven.

The Bible also speaks of heaven being filled with streets of gold. I imagine heaven as being a place of joy. That was what I experienced that day, I was at peace.

Before we get to what I consider a key time in my life I have to introduce you to 2 other people that have become dear friends. Jaime McNab and Charla Valenzuela. Jaime and Charla are cousins. They are also amazing leaders and are people you can lean on when times are tough. They are wise beyond measure. Jaime introduced me to Advocare. She had

observed me when we attended Geyer Springs
Baptist Church. She was well aware of the
struggles endured with my health. Jaime
reached out to me with an opportunity to put
something in my life, which at the time I didn't
completely understand how much it would later
benefit me. Jaime cared enough to share
something with me that would eventually unlock
the door to the current season of my life.

Charla is one tough cookie. She isn't
afraid to look you in the face and tell you how it
is. Charla is our diamond leader in our
Advocare organization. She used to be a coach
and isn't afraid to tell you that you have a
problem and need to do something.

And that is where we pick up with this
journey. I remember it well, we had a spark

mixer and Charla was there. Afterward, we were just hanging around talking. Charla looked me in the face and asked me one question followed with a statement which is seared on my mind. "What is your health worth to you?" No one had ever asked me a question like this. But what got me even more was her follow up statement. Charla told me if I didn't do something, I could forget seeing my girls get married let alone graduate from high school.

That hit hard. It was at that very moment I began searching for my heart and earnestly seeking God's guidance. I knew deep down inside something had to change, I just didn't know how.

Fast forward to April 2017. The weeks leading up to the crossroads of my health and wellness, were extremely nerve-wracking. My primary care doctor referred me to CARTI for what initially was a blood abnormality. My doctor eventually wanted to do a CT scan. The morning of the CT scan I also had a sleep study consultation.

When I arrived at the consultation my vital check revealed an oxygen level of 78%. I spent six days in the hospital before I was actually scheduled for my sleep study. Results of the sleep study led to a diagnosis of sleep apnea. Not long after my sleep study, the results of the CT scan revealed a golf ball size lymph node in my left groin. A biopsy revealed there was no cancer was revealed.

While in the hospital, I prayed daily for God to restore my health. I firmly believe the result of that biopsy was the moment God started restoring my health. He was answering my prayer for him to restore my health. God started to reveal to me the things I needed to change for the process to work. My mindset started to change. The way I saw the food in my mouth changed, my energy increased which resulted in me being able to move easier without feeling wiped out. You see I learned that I had a problem and I had to deal with it. Rather than looking for what I thought was a solution I had to come to the understand I had a serious problem and if I didn't take the right action, I would be right back at square one.

During those days in the hospital, I prayed a lot. I mean, when you're in the hospital and you are mainly in for observation, with not a lot of visitors that's about the only thing you can do. I prayed the same prayer each day, for God to restore my health. It became a constant theme for my prayers not only during my hospital stay but also the days after. It was then, God started to reveal to me what I needed to change for this journey to even be possible.

I was already taking amazing nutritional supplements from advocare, so my metabolism primed and ready for the journey. My boat was in the water and the motor was ready to run, I just needed to change the fuel.

Before April of 2017, I wasn't taking my nutrition and exercise seriously. I truly believe had the hospital stay not happened, I would have probably hit 500 pounds in no time. With the increase in my energy, I had a strong desire to exercise and get to moving. Because of the changes, I made with my nutrition, combined with the exercise I was doing, and the supplements I was using my journey to better health and a better life was beginning to take shape. I also believe that hospital stay drew me closer to God. I have a better understanding of God's healing power and why he is the great physician. I firmly believe that God heard my prayers and began to stir in me something amazing.

My exercise consisted of riding one to two miles a day, 4 days a week. I started tracking my weight loss and after my first week I had dropped 8 pounds. That was huge! My confidence started to grow. The weight loss journey was on. 2 miles a day would soon grow

17

to 5 miles a day, then 7, and eventually 10 miles a day. Now, anything below 15 miles a day is a disappointment to me. I continue to set my standard high, so I have something to achieve each and every time I get on my bicycle for a ride.

I also took part in 2 different gladiator challenges. I started adding more strength training. I learned how to use a nutrition macro, so I could track my nutrition on a daily basis. Using a nutrition macro helps to hold you accountable. By the time I finished the first 6-week challenge, I had gone from 453 pounds to around 390 pounds. I also received the title, master gladiator.

During June 2017, I participated in the Great American Cycle Challenge, a fund-raising event for Children's Cancer Research. My goal was to raise $500 and ride 50 miles. I met both goals and received an awesome cycling jersey. I backed that up a year later in June of 2018 with a 243-mile month, more than breaking my 200-mile goal for the 2018 Great Cycle Challenge and I raised $579 for Children's Cancer Research. Having these goals made me think about how much weight I wanted to lose. I really started to believe that a realistic goal would be to get down to 250 pounds. The more I see success on the scale, the more I realize that goal was attainable. I just had to work hard and fight every day.

Cycling has been my primary form of exercising. I have had some amazing moments when God spoke to me while I was riding. A reminder he will always be by my side no matter

what I face in life.

The Desire to Fight Like a Gladiator

Setting out on a journey requires fighting hard and doing the little things. If you look at what a gladiator used as his weapons or tools for battle, you have to begin to think of what you need to help you along your journey as you battle to see successes and reach your goals.

One of the primary weapons used by the gladiator is the sword. The word of God is just that for me. My Bible is my two-edged sword. Not only is obesity a physical battle, but it is also a spiritual battle. Satan tries to throw doubt in your way and tries to make you think that you can't do it. Philippians 4:13, "For I can do all things through Christ who strengthens me." With God anything is possible.

Not only did gladiators use a sword or in some cases a bow and arrow, but they also had protection in the form of a shield and a helmet, and armor for their arms and legs. From the spiritual aspect, my relationship with God is like that armor. He is my shield and protector. With weight loss, you must have things that will help protect you along the journey, so you don't regress. This protection takes on what I believe are four basic pillars of successful weight loss and put you in a better position to maintain the end goal whether its 20 pounds or 200 pounds.

Successful weight loss starts with the most basic tool, sleep. You have to sleep well at night. Not getting enough sleep you will have a hard time functioning and in turn, will lack the energy to build a foundation of support for the other pillars of successful weight loss. For me, I was lucky to get 3 hours of sleep. Late nights made it difficult to fall asleep which lead to staying away one to two hours. Lack of sleep lead to feeling miserable and tired. There were days at work I would fall asleep

The next tool for successful weight loss is the need to change bad nutrition habits. It is important to fuel our bodies with proper nutrition. Replacing bad habits with better nutritional choices will make a positive impact on your health and wellness. Remember the old adage, garbage in garbage out. If I'm putting junk in my body, it will respond in a negative way. If I'm putting healthy food in my body, it will respond in a positive way.

I would eat at Rally's and Taco Bell no less than three days a week. I was stuck in a rut. It was cheap and easy to drive through, pick up, and take back to work. My medical bills started piling up as a result of my poor nutrition habits. Maybe, eating fast food and junk wasn't so cheap after all. Since I changed my nutrition choices and have lost my weight I haven't had to worry about medical bills because I haven't had to go back in the hospital because of my poor choices. So, that means not only has my physical health improved but so has our financial health.

The third pillar needed for successful weight loss is exercise. You have to move and be motivated to move. If you exercise 30 minutes to an hour a day you will see weight loss success. Initially, I was so sluggish because of my poor eating habits and health that it was difficult to even exercise 15 minutes. My knees hurt, and I was gasping for air in a matter of minutes.

After I was diagnosed with sleep apnea and put on a machine to help me sleep better, I started getting a sudden boost of energy. With a boost in energy came a desire to move. What did it look like for me? About a year or two before my hospital stay, April 2017, I had purchased a Trek Shift hybrid bicycle. The only problem, it was collecting dust and was becoming a waste of money. So, I decided to start riding it. Even if it was only 30 minutes or 1 mile it didn't matter.

The beginning of any weight loss journey should start with changing eating habits. Exercise is important. When everything is working in concert, there will be results. I did, and my confidence level started increasing. But remember, exercise doesn't mean going to the gym and trying to bench press 500 pounds. Even a walk around the block a couple of times will help. Remember, the key to exercise is moving and getting those steps in.

The final pillar for successful weight loss is the use of multivitamins and nutritional supplements. Having a strong supplement program to help kick-start your metabolism is important. A year ago, I was obese and my metabolism slow. It needed to be primed.

My supplements of choice come from Advocare. Advocare offers world-class products that are safe and add value to my life. When Jamie McNab introduced me to Advocare, I was skeptical. While I saw other people using supplements and protein powders, those people were already pretty fit. At 400 plus pounds, I didn't see supplements as something beneficial. Not to mention, our financial situation at the time. That's when Jamie showed me how I could get a discount on my products.

First, I started off with a 24-day jumpstart. I was very inconsistent, and that inconsistency showed. But after the face to face with Charla, I started doing some soul searching and just came to the conclusion something had to give. I had to get my life and health back in

27

order even if it meant cutting something out to be able to afford what I knew was the key to getting my journey back on track then so be it. And a few weeks afterward I was back in the hospital for what was my last major hospital stay in 2 years.

Here is why I believe proper supplementation is important. Even with the food we eat, we still face nutritional shortfalls. The only way to fill the void is with the right supplements. Now, I do think there are some people who go overboard with supplements and probably take things they aren't going to benefit from. I have found the right combination that gives me daily multivitamins, protein, and carbs. With the combination eating right and exercise, it has been the blueprint for successful weight loss.

The whole key is allowing these pillars to work in concert. Once everything in place, successful weight loss that is sustainable and easy to maintain. And that's what this journey is all about for me, the desire and passion to add value to my life but not just my life. I want to be able to add value to my wife, my daughters, and anyone else willing to step out of their comfort zone and start their own journey to a new person. I am passionate about sharing my story with others, not so I can seek fame and fortune but, so I can add value and make a difference in the lives of other people. Just like other people have walked the journey with me, I too want to return the favor.

If there is one thing I have learned on this journey, my success has been possible because I've added things of value. So, what exactly does this mean? I've surrounded myself with other people who encourage and push me to succeed. These people correct when I screw up and teach me how to improve the process. I've also replaced things that drag me down with things that build me up. My bicycle, for example, has added value to my life. The more I ride the better I get. The more I ride the further I am able to ride. Because of this, my confidence has gone up. When I was over 450 pounds I lacked confidence. I had a mindset that I couldn't do what I am doing now. So as my confidence has gone up, I have started moving beyond just riding for exercise to walking, more strength training, and even an occasional boot camp class.

The supplements I take also add value to my life. I've seen my blood sugar level remain in a normal range. Which, in turn, helped me to come off one insulin and close to coming off my other insulin. My story is an example of what is possible if you do it the right way. I believe my story will add value to the lives of others.

Chase Your Medal

Running a marathon often means chasing a medal or trophy of some kind. I competed in my first two 5K's this last year. The second of these 5K's was part of the 2018 Little Rock Marathon weekend. The Little Rock Marathon awards finishers medals to everyone who completes the 5K or any other event they participate in that weekend. The idea of completing the 5K was a huge accomplishment to me, but also chasing after the medal drove me to take each step along the route until I completed the course no matter how long it took.

But just like a 5K or marathon there are medals I chase after on a daily basis. My weight loss is important not only for me but for my family. The medal I am chasing after is the 250-

pound mark. The cool thing about it, I can do it. With God having my back and in control, I know I can. He has been working in my life to release me from the bondage of obesity. He is restoring my health. This is the reason I am driven to my passion to help other people chase their medal.

The question to be asked, what does that medal look like for you? Is it about losing a few inches or pounds? Is it about getting healthy? For me, it was about getting healthy for my family. Look at the concept of chasing the medal like you would goal setting. Set your goals and chase after them. In order to achieve those goals, you have to set your standard high. Chase after those goals with reckless abandon. When you're in a desperate situation like I was, have the mentality that to fight and chase at all

costs. Look at goals as an incentive to stay the

course and be committed to the process.

When I first started on this journey the

one food I completely cut out of my nutrition

choices was beef, yes beef. I needed to eat clean

and lean proteins. So, I vowed not to eat another

steak until I got below 250 pounds. I guess you

could say that steak dinner is my marathon

medal for this unbelievable weight loss journey.

Believe me, the steak dinner will be the best I

have ever had. Not only was a steak dinner a

goal I set, but I also set goals along the way

related to my fitness accomplishments. And of

course, I set smaller weight loss goals to

accomplish until I reach my ultimate number of

200 pounds lost. So, set your goals but make

them attainable.

Questions That Have to Be Answered Honestly

When I started my process, there were several questions that I was asked or just ran through my mind. If not now when? When you're faced with a crisis in life and something has to change what is holding you back? Why are you letting whatever that is keep you from deciding on better health?

These are the questions I had to answer. When I first started with AdvoCare some 4 to 5 years ago I was asked what my health was worth to me. It really didn't hit me until I was in the hospital in April of 2017. I was tired of having to be admitted to the hospital for things which could be avoided simply by changing how I was eating and by exercising. I saw my health as being worth far more than the debt from medical bills. I have a wife and two precious daughters who need me. Even when I wasn't in the hospital, feeling sluggish and always hurting wholesale changes were needed. No amount of money will equal being able to walk 2 miles while your children ride their bikes. Being able to hear your wife say how she feels to wrap her arms around you when she gives you a hug is worth so much more than all the medical debt I have had over the last 12 years.

I answered these questions honestly, and decided a healthy life was a no-brainer. Money was just an excuse. I had to stop making excuses and think about how much my health was worth. If you're like me, you have people in your life who mean the world to you. So when you are faced with a decision involving your health and wellness you also have to think about those people closest to you. Who are you changing for? As a father and a husband, I had to make sure I was in a better position to be around for my family. When you're faced with a health crisis which requires you to make wholesale changes, you'll do whatever it takes to see successful weight loss, so you are around for those people who mean the most to you.

Being honest with yourself means you have to realize you have problems. Once you realize you have problems, you then have to find solutions to those problems. A prime example of this would be if you had a slow leak in a tire. You have to be able to identify where the leak is before you can repair it or if it is even possible to repair the tire. Once you realize you have a problem, you can then explore ways to solve the problem. But don't wait until its too late. As soon as you identify your problem take action, don't let it fester until you end up as I did 13 years ago when I was diagnosed with type 2 diabetes or 2 years ago when I was back in the hospital with a low oxygen issue. It all goes back to staying in tune to life.

Being in Bondage to Obesity

If you've ever heard of Celebrate Recovery you would probably associate it with someone who is a recovering alcoholic or drug addict. This is far from the truth. In fact, Celebrate Recovery or any other ministry like this is for anyone who is in bondage to something. What it looks like for one person to the next may not be the same.

To be in bondage to something means whatever that something is, has a stronghold of over your life. It also means you aren't doing anything to allow God to break the chains and free you from that bondage. Obesity is no different. Being in bondage means being in denial of a problem. That's where I was for many years. It didn't matter what my parents, wife, or friends would say because I didn't see it as a problem. I thought I was overweight because it was hereditary or because it was how God made me. I'm 45 years old, I haven't been obese my entire life. As a matter of fact, I have probably only weighed over 300 pounds in the last 15 years of my life.

How did I get to be at that point in my life? I ate junk, I ate fast food at least 3 days a week and sometime 5 days a week. Fast food was easier than taking the time to prepare meals at home. My food choices included, pizza, cokes, sweet tea, and anything fried. So, what led to obesity all goes back to choices. This is no different than anything else I could be in bondage to. The choices eventually led to the life-changing health experience I described

41

earlier. These were the consequences of those poor choices I continued to make. I have vowed not to spend time in the hospital because of a poor choice I made.

Last April when I was in the hospital God began to stir in my heart the need to change. Something had to change and that's when God began breaking the chains that held me in bondage. I prayed daily for God to restore my health. I firmly believe he heard my prayer and has answered. God began to release me from the bondage of obesity. I started making better choices with my food. I have learned to meal prep, which makes it easier to know what I am putting in my mouth. I started seeing a boost in my energy level. With the increase in my energy, I had a strong desire to exercise. With

42

the combination of better nutritional concepts and a strong exercise regimen, I started seeing results immediately. Which is what this is all about, results. Results early on were losing 5 to 6 pounds a week. Results now are seeing my body fat percent drop 8% in 4 months and my muscle weight increase by 8 pounds. Results now also mean my body composition change. Once you see results, your confidence will increase, and you will know that if you set your mind and heart to it and allow God to move in your life he will break you free from the bondage of obesity.

Dig Roots and Grow

When I refer to digging roots, I believe that is where growth begins to take hold. When a seed is planted, roots begin to sprout before the plant comes out of the ground. Sometimes the process may take days, weeks, or even months for that plant to even appear. The same can be said for weight loss. It has to start somewhere, and somewhere means making the decision to commit to a healthy lifestyle. You didn't put the weight on overnight and it definitely won't come off overnight. Once you have come to the point where you've decided to make the commitment and begin to make the necessary changes to lose the weight, then it's time to grow. My roots start with my relationship with God. I firmly believe having that relationship with God is important because of what He adds to life. He provides rich soil for me to grow in. Without Him in my life, it would be like trying to plant a garden on rocky ground, you can forget getting anything to grow. Then there's my family, from my parents, Vernon and Geneva Crow to my wife and girls. Finally, my advocare family is the fertilizer that has helped to keep the process going.

Growing means doing everything it takes to see results. Just like my walk with God, results are the equivalent to the fruit you bear through your relationship with God and how you live your life. My growth has come from different sources. The main source has been my relationship with God, reading the Bible and spending time with him. Surrounding myself with other people who have been there to cheer

me on and offer words of encouragement.

Those things are important for growth. Without

them, you would wither away like the garden the

gardener failed to tend to. So, remember, dig

roots and grow.

Locked into Life

One of the outlets which I enjoy is cycling. I have been riding for over a year now. When I first started riding, I used standard pedals and wore regular tennis shoes. Anyone who follows cycling knows the best way to increase your performance on the bike is to use clipless pedals and shoes that clip into the pedals.

When I am clipped in, I'm able to utilize all my complete muscle group. But as I have been thinking about being clipped in on my bike, it reminds me so much about life and how you have to be focused on a daily basis in all aspects of your life. Cycling is no different.

When I am clipped into my pedals I must understand when to slow down. I have to

47

pay attention to everyone else. When you get to that point, you have to know the appropriate time to unclip. If I unclip to soon ay a high rate of speed I could wreck. No clipping in fast enough, could lead to me falling over and getting hurt. The sound of something breaking on my bike means it's time to stop and check it out. There might be a flat, broken chain, or a spoke could have popped.

Life is no different, it is important to understand when to slow down, to avoid overdoing it. Understanding the queues your body gives. It may be time to stop and refocus. Pay more attention to what is truly important.

Especially with your health, you have to pay attention to different signs. When someone is having chest pains and an arm is hurting, it is time to go to the doctor. Headaches and breathing problems are also cause for concern. The point is, continually doing the same thing over and over again and not making the necessary changes to see successful weight loss will not lead to improved health and wellness. Eating right, exercising, and maybe even adding nutritional supplements fill in the nutrition gap. Once the right path is chosen, stay focused. But remember, it is ok to fall. One of the things I have learned with cycling is when I have to stop for something whether it is for a drink of water or an issue with my bike, other cyclists will stop and make sure I am ok. In life, I must surround myself with other people who will be an encouragement and pick me up when I fall.

Being locked into all aspects of life improve my

chances of living a long healthy life.

Commit to be Consistent

When you arrive at a point in your life where you have to lose weight it is important to remember it's a process. The process can take time and requires commitment. Becoming overweight does not magically happen overnight. And it will only come off if I stay the course. When you are overweight like I have been, you have to remember that the weight didn't magically appear overnight. To see the weight come off you have to stay the course. This is what it means to be consistent. It's this way with anything in your life. Consistency means stability, stability means standing on a firm foundation. Having a firm foundation is important because it means you are less likely to waver or get off course.

So, what does it mean to commit to being consistent? In terms of health and wellness, as stated before, it is a process. For me, that process starts at the beginning of the week prepping my meals for the upcoming week. Meal prep is important because I know every ingredient that goes into each of my meals. Whereas if I went out to eat lunch every day how am I supposed to know what is in the food I eat? Simply put, I have no idea what was used to prepare that fast food or junk I just purchased. Meal prepping combined with use of a fitness and nutrition app keeps me honest and holds me accountable as I am able to track my daily food intake.

Another part of the process involves nutritional supplements and vitamins. These are necessary to fill any nutritional gaps I have with the food I eat. You'll start to feel better, in turn feeling better about yourself. You'll feel better emotionally and physically.

Finally, you have to exercise at least 30 minutes a day, 6 days a week. Exercise will get metabolism revved up and going. Being able to speed metabolism up will go a long way toward burning calories and in turn, will see lead to weight loss. Proper exercise mixes a combination of cardio with resistance training. Resistance training is important in order to build muscle mass. Gaining more muscle mass makes it easier to keep the fat off, making muscles lean, I exercise 30 minutes a day, 6 days a week.

Looking back on Dig Roots and Grow, being consistent is all a part of the growing part.

At times pruning out the weeds. Weeds

represent the small things that may not work.

Pruning is needed to continue growing. The

more growth, the easier it becomes to stay

consistent with the process.

Revisiting My Purpose

It is important to know and understand your purpose. My journey over the last year has opened my eyes to the seriousness of obesity. So many people are obese, to the point of serious health issues. Case in point, I have lived with type 2 diabetes for the last 12 years of my life. Only over the last year have I been able to see improvements in my health. This epidemic, if you will, can be defeated if people learn to change their habits and make better choices. Many of the health issues associated with obesity can then be avoided. This is why I believe my purpose involves helping other people, struggling as I have for so long, get their weight under control in a manner that is responsible and sustainable.

My heart breaks when I see someone else struggle to walk five feet because they're so overweight they lose their breath. My heart breaks when I see someone in this situation who continues making the same choices over and over again with no desire to change. My passion is to walk hand in hand, locked arms, on the same journey I have been in the last year or so. I have a desire to see people realize a new healthy lifestyle is possible if they just make the commitment and chase after that prize.

My purpose is also in my relationship with God. He is that firm foundation that gives me the standing I need to see the change I have seen in my health and wellness. I firmly believe that he is restoring my health for one reason, and that is the way I started each day while I was in the hospital last year. I prayed specifically for God to restore my health. I believe in the power of prayer.

I also believe in the importance of being an example for others to follow. 1 Timothy 4:12, "Let no one despise you for your youth, but set the believers an example in speech, in conduct, in love, in purity." Every time I hear someone say that my story is an inspiration to them, I want to strive daily to be the right example. An example to help others reach their goals involving health and wellness. Inspiring others means so much more than winning a transformation competition. When I can play a part in helping someone see significant weight loss and reach their health goals, that make this journey I'm on worthwhile.

From Feeling Old & Sluggish to Young & Vibrant

When I weighed 453 pounds It was so hard to get around without feeling like I was out of breath or about to pass out. Think about your car when you need an oil change or add air to a tire, but you put it off so long that your car starts to run sluggish and that tire wears out so much that it is bald and there is no tread left on the tire. Well, this is exactly how I felt, so when you get that oil changed or those new tires man, your car runs much better and drives much smoother.

Losing weight is no different. The more you lose, the better you start to feel. I know for me I don't feel sluggish anymore and my knees don't hurt like they once did. The key going forward is being able to maintain what I've been

58

doing. It is no different than your car maintenance. For your car to run right you have to stay on a regular maintenance schedule. With your health and wellness, you have to maintain what you are doing so you don't regress and start to gain the weight back. As you do what is necessary to lose weight and maintain that weight loss you will feel better all the time. Who doesn't want to feel better?

I may be 45 years old, but I feel like I'm 10 years younger. I feel like I've gone from a Lincoln town car to Shelby Mustang. I can walk a mile, whereas before I could barely walk five feet. I can ride 3 miles on my bike at 13 miles per hour. Before I could barely ride 1 mile. I can get out and walk while my girls ride their bikes and I can keep up with them. Before I had a hard time keeping up.

Not only am I cycling but I have been walking more this year. I have walked in three 5k's over the last year. I did a great inflatable race with my girls. I walked 2 miles in the Rocket 5k. My youngest daughter, Bailey, walked in Great Strides for Cystic Fibrosis. I rode 200 miles during the month of June. I mention these events because a year ago none of this would have been possible because of the shape I was in. because I've allowed God to have complete control of my life my drive to do more is so much stronger. The more I walk, the longer the distance I ride, the more my confidence increases. With the support of my wife and so many friends, I have no doubt I'll cross the finish line and see my weight below

250 pounds.

The Finish Line

Whether a 5k or a 30-mile cycling event, as you approach the finish line there are people there cheering you on. In many cases, there are people along the route cheering you on. When you cross the finish line there's a sense of completion. There is also a sense of accomplishment. You're excited that you just received a medal.

The more I ride and walk in various walking or cycling events, my confidence increases. The more I lose weight I have the confidence to keep going and not stop until I cross the finish line. Every time I do a 5k or ride a cycling event I set a goal to finish and finish strong. When I set the goal to lose 200 pounds, I did so with the mindset to finish strong.

When I cross the finish line I'll have a sense of accomplishment. My wife and other family and friends will be there cheering me on and celebrate when I cross the 250-pound finish line. It won't be about where I started, rather it will be about how I finished.

This Journey to 250 pounds has had its challenges. Any journey will have mountain top highs and valley lows. They key is how to respond when faced with adversity. Push through the obstacles that get in the way. Along the way, I have come up with some catchphrases such as commit to be consistent or dig roots and grow. As you're on your journey you have to push forward with determination. What that means is you have to do it no matter what you face. The more you do it the easier it will be and will eventually become natural because it has been engraved into the fabric of your life. The less you stop making excuses and find ways to get beyond the obstacles reaching your goal will be well worth the push and determination. Next thing you know, you're within reach of the finish line and people will be there cheering you on until the finish. When you reach the finish line and cross it that will be the most rewarding accomplishment you will have ever achieved. It's like a medal you received when you complete a 5k or marathon. The day I walked in the Little Rock 5k, I received a medal when I crossed the finish line. Receiving the medal gave me a sense of accomplishment I just achieved something that a year earlier would have been nearly impossible. That's how a weight loss journey is. So, fight on with the determination of a mule. Why a mule? Mules are stubborn and determined to do what they want no matter what.

The After Party

Now that I have lost weight, what next? I have to maintain what I've lost. That's how weight loss is. Once you get to the desired weight, you have to do what it takes to maintain that weight.

This is also how it is supposed to be as a Christian. When you are saved you have to do the necessary things to grow as a believer in God and not just remain stagnant in your faith. That starts with reading your bible and praying each and every day of the week. You also have to surround yourself with other believers. When you do these things and allow God to have complete control, a journey like the one I have been on is so much easier to deal with.

66

My journey is similar to cycling. When you start out on the journey you have so much to learn. The same can be said for cycling. The more you do it, the easier it becomes. As you progress in cycling you develop skills that make certain feats easier to take on. With the journey I am on to better health I have learned so many new things along the way that have done nothing but improve my health and help me get to a point where sustaining the weight will become much easier. But with cycling, there will come a time when the only way to improve your skills, you have to clip into your pedals. At that point it takes razor-sharp focus, so you don't make a mistake and fall over. When you are on a journey to better health you have got to remember to be focused and if you ever fall pick

67

yourself up and keep going. And remember,

surround yourself with other people who can and

will be your support and offer encouragement

along the way. When you achieve your health

goals you have to be an inspiration for others

who struggle daily as they live in bondage to

obesity. Do that and one person at a time we

will be able to defeat obesity.

Be Locked into Life

Through everything I have learned on my journey the one thing that probably sums it all up is the need to be locked into life. What does that mean? As I think back to 13 years ago when I was diagnosed with diabetes and had the pulmonary embolism. For the first couple of years I became in tuned to pains which were similar to what I experienced leading up to the embolism. If there was even a hint of similar pain in my legs I was calling the doctor and going for an MRI to make sure I did not have another blood clot. Leading up to the pulmonary embolism, I really wasn't tuned into all the signs that something serious was about to happen to me. I was sick with headaches all the time, I was sick with colds and bronchitis. Those

69

should have been signs I should have paid close attention to, but I blew them off and kept living life how I saw fit.

Fast forward to April 2017 when I had the low oxygen issue that put me back in the hospital for yet another extended stay. The signs of sleep apnea were there, but I put it off to the point where I had to be admitted to the hospital for observation and eventually a sleep study.

You have to be in tune to what is going on at all times, so you will be able to respond in a way that will get you the help you need to overcome setbacks. Weight loss is no different, you are going to have setbacks along the way if you aren't focused and locked into what is going on. If you stay locked into everything you face on a daily basis you will be able to adjust your journey accordingly. This means it is important to allow for flexibility, so you can overcome the setbacks. Having flexibility will let you adjust, so you are able to avoid the pitfalls along the path.

In terms of health and wellness, it takes 80 days to form a habit. It also takes 1 day to break the habit. So, what does it mean? You can work hard for 30 days and have one day where you get off course, next thing you know you have started to gain the weight back because you have started to make bad habits again. So being locked into a life and what is happening along the path will help you avoid breaking those good habits you have formed and are forming on the weight loss journey. You have to realize, there will be days you might not feel much like getting in 30 minutes of exercise, you

might pass by that fast food restaurant that

allows for an easy in and out with your supper

for the night. Those are the kinds of things

which can unravel all the hard work you put in

to get to the point you are, you don't want to let

those things keep you from reaching your

ultimate goal.

Base, Push, All Out

I recently started working out, two days a week, at Orange Theory Fitness. The workouts are intense. They offer a great mix of cardio and strength. What makes Orange Theory unique is the three phases they use-base, push, and all-out. Thinking about those phases, it hit me how they can be used as an analogy to describe the weight loss journey.

Let's first start by taking a look at the base pace. The way I view this phase in terms of weight loss, this is your starting point. There has to be a launch point in order for the process to even begin. What does this look like? For some, it may be something as simple as changing the way you eat or just exercising 30 minutes a day. For others, it may require

73

wholesale changes. But those changes shouldn't be too extreme. Going all out too fast and not seeing results leads to loss in confidence. So, the base pace is where your foundation is built. Once that foundation has become solidified, it's time to get out of your comfort zone and begin to push to the next level of the process.

The push phase is where subtle changes take place. Clothes start to fit different, your body composition change, and most importantly your confidence begins to increase. Stepping out of your comfort zone and start exploring the better your chances of sticking to the process. There may be times where change is needed. Try exercise or nutrition to give your system a jolt.

Once you've gotten through the plateau, it's time to step up your game. This is where the all-out phase comes into play. This phase is uncomfortable. Look for extraordinary things to do so you reach the ultimate weight loss goal. This may involve lowering caloric intake to trim the last bit of fat off your belly. It may mean trying something like keto, long enough to get the last bit of fat trimmed off. Maybe challenge yourself in the gym or with the at- home exercise routine. Instead of walking 2 miles a day walk 4. Instead of doing 30 minutes on the bike trainer, go an hour. Doing these extra things may seem a bit much but remember, the end result will be the most rewarding.

Before reaching the final results, chisel away the imperfections. I like to watch the TV show, Gold Rush. I am amazed at the process

they use to catch gold. Starting with digging the

pay dirt to hauling it to the wash plant. But

that's only part of the process. Once the rocks

have been washed and the mats pulled there's all

this concentrate that still has to be washed in a

smaller version of the wash plant. The gold is

separated from what dirt there is, revealing a

beautiful shiny piece of metal worth so much per

ounce. That's kind of how the weight loss

process is. You have to get rid of the fat through

diet, exercise, and proper supplementation

before you can even get to what's underneath

the fat. That's the fun thing about the process.

Seeing the muscle definition and veins

becoming more vascular, you'll start to gain a

better understanding of what your body has gone

through to reach this point. You will understand that once you reach that point, keeping it off and maintaining it will be so much easier to do than if your weight starts to roller coaster. You have to do what works for you. Remember, your journey will be amazing, especially once you reach the ultimate prize. So find a base to build from, push forward, and go all out.

Seeing is Believing

The amazing thing about losing weight is going back to the beginning and seeing the transformation my body has gone through. I would like to share my transformation pictures, so you are able to see with your own eyes what this journey has been about for me.

Me at 453 pounds

This is when my weight loss journey began.

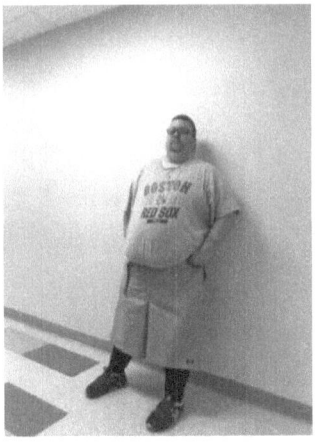

Slim & Trim 2019

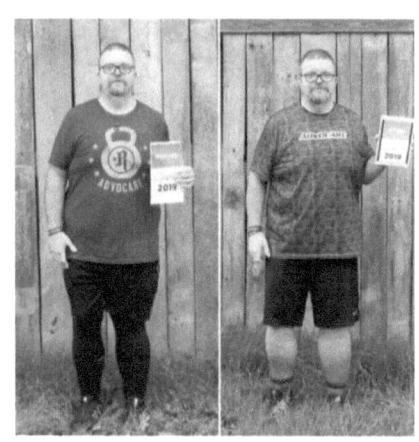

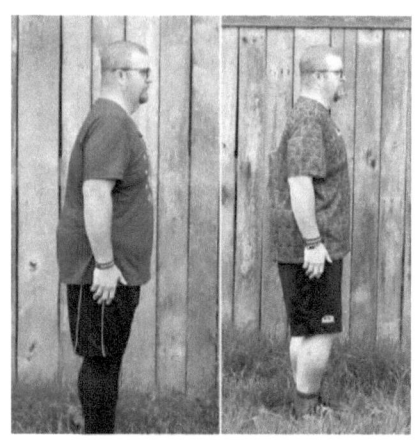

Big Dam Bridge 100

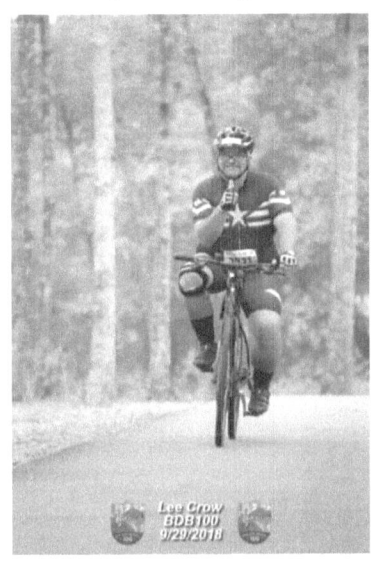

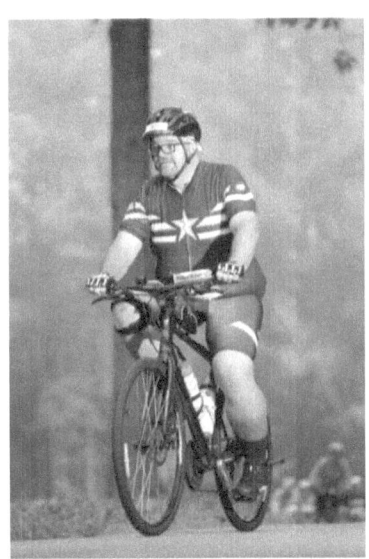

Tour De Rock 2019

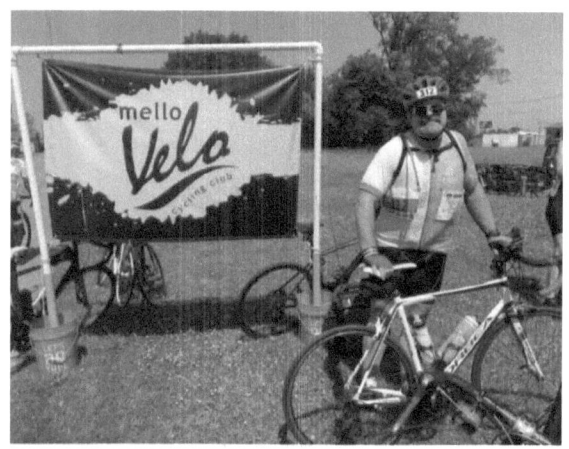

2018 Little Rock 5K

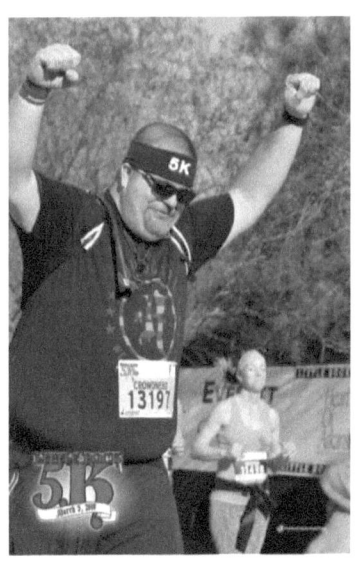

2019 Little Rock 10K

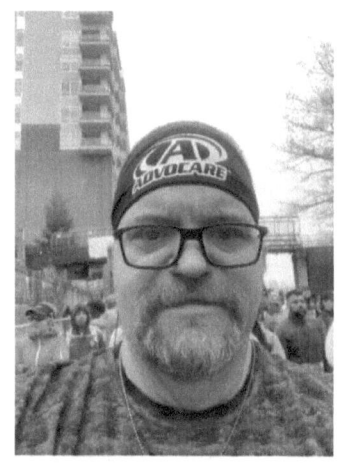

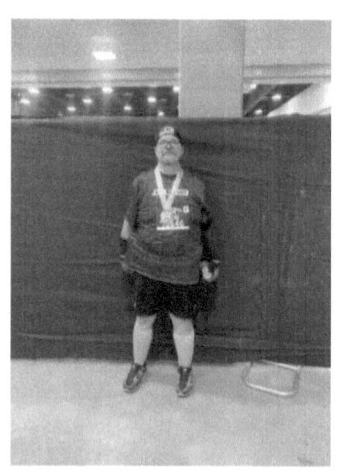

The idea of seeing is believing is extremely important. Being able to look back on the images and shows how everything— physically and emotionally has changed. Not only will other people be able to see the changes, if they too are struggling with their weight it will give a sense of hope. They will see it is possible to overcome the weight issues, get it off, and live a normal healthy life. That is why I decided to write this book.

So, as you lose weight get hold of your transformation images so you can look back on the journey from beginning to end so you can be amazed at the difference you made in your own life. It gives you a sense of pride and helps build your own confidence. Someone who is overweight, and struggles has a hard time with their confidence, I know this all too well because I was there. If I had a hard time doing something because of my weigh I had zero confidence I could do it. When weight started coming off my confidence level increased. It all goes back to something I mentioned earlier in the book, you have to change how you think and feel before you can even begin to see the results. That's why it is so important to make sure you are putting the right foods in your mouth and not eating junk.

If you are struggling or know something struggling this book was written with them in mind to show them there are people who can relate. My prayer is to see obesity eradicated. The only way this will be possible is for people to get on the journey and stay on it because

living a healthy lifestyle is just that, a lifestyle.

It is a way of life for me, let it be a way of life

for you too. From spiritual wellbeing to health

and wellness. From feeding the mind and heart

to feeding stomach. It all has an effect. Do you

want to have negativity in your life or do you

want to live at peace? Follow the process and

stick to it. You will be able to live a healthy life

and be at peace knowing that your old way of

living, with the struggles associated with

obesity, will no longer be part of your life.

That's the hope I have for myself as well as

other people struggling with weight. A hope we

be at peace knowing that we have turned from

the struggles and are able to live life knowing

our health and wellness is the best it has ever

been.

God, Family, Friends

When I first introduced you to my family and friends. I did so to show the importance of having a strong support group. That support starts with a firm foundation. For me, that foundation is grounded in my relationship with God. You see, I have had a relationship with God since I was 19 years old. Have I always lived perfect, of course not, I am an imperfect man who serves a perfect God. He has and will always be by my side. With that firm foundation, it is also necessary to have a supportive family.

Without family support it is difficult to face challenges in life. Which is why I am thankful first for a wife who has stood by me when she could have easily pulled her tent stakes and walked out. It is also important to have a strong relationship with your children and be in tune to them each and every day. You never know what you will learn from them that can be applied to your situation. And then my parents, while to some it may not be cool to still have parents involved even at my age, but you know, I am thankful to have parents who are still living and am able to spend quality time with them. It's that quality time which helps push me to continue fighting on this journey because I want to be at my healthiest when I am in my 70's.

Then there are my friends. While I named Charla and Jamie earlier, I have so many friends who have played a vital role along my journey. One friend I have yet to mention is

Fred Dickson. I consider Fred my cycling mentor. We used to work together. Fred has taught me so much not just about cycling but about life. One thing I have learned from him is patience. Because when you cycle, there are times you have to be patient. Just like with weight loss you have to be patient because there will be weeks when you are going to lose 1 pound or no weight at all. Fred has also taught me the importance of considering other factors when riding. The same can be said with weight loss.

Another important reason it is important to have strong support from friends also involves my love for cycling. I joined the Mello Velo Cycling club in 2018. One of my last rides of 2018 was a ride I will never forget. I was riding with some friends and had my first and so far only fall on my bike. We were on the last leg of the ride, riding through downtown Little Rock. I got caught up on some trolley tracks. One of the first things you will learn when cycling, is never get parallel to tracks. Well, in this case, I had no choice because of the road we were on at the time. The problem I ran into, I was in the middle of the track rather than to the outside. An attempt to cross over led to my front tire getting caught, throwing me from the bike. Here's where the importance of friends comes into play. The people riding with me, Carol, Stephanie, and Edwin all helped me get up and made sure I was ok. I was able to get back on my bike and finish the ride. I mention this because when you have hard weeks on the weight loss journey, you have to have someone there to help pick you up and encourage you. The encouragement helps build confidence and helps get you to a point where you can overcome those weeks when you get easily discouraged and frustrated. Believe me when I say, you will experience those weeks. You just can't give up. You have to keep pushing forward.

Meet My Family

This is Amanda Michelle Crow, she is my rock. She has stuck by my side through this entire journey, all the way back to when I was diagnosed with diabetes. We have been married 17 years. I met her at a time in my life I never thought I would get married. Boy was I wrong.

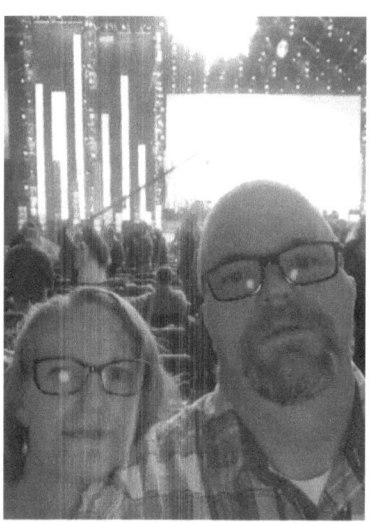

These are my girls when they were babies. Bethany is our miracle from God. She has taught us so much about overcoming obstacles. She never ceases to amaze us when she accomplishes something, we never thought possible. Bailey is our second miracle. She is always keeping us on our toes and has those times when she has meltdown and needs a hug to help her get through it.

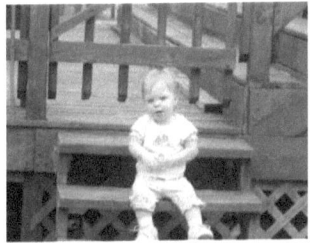

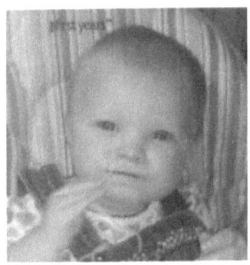

Here I am with my girls at the 2019
Great Inflatable Race. It is times like these,
where I am reminded exactly what it is I am
fighting for. These girls were amazing during
this time we had together.

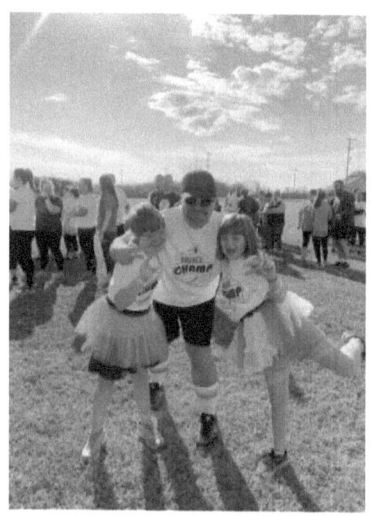

Reaching My 200 Pound Goal

When I set out on this journey, I set a goal to lose 200 pounds. I recently hit that goal. When I first started out, I weighed a whopping 453 pounds. On May 22, 2019, I stepped on the scaled three times and each time I saw the number 253 show up. I've always heard the saying, third times the charm. Well, I tend to agree. This was the greatest feeling in the world, knowing I achieved a 2-year goal that I set at the beginning of my journey. While there were several small goals that I reached along the journey, this goal means the most. This goal represents the stick and stay mentality I have developed. It means that I stuck to the process. It means that I can accomplish anything that I set my mind to. These 2 years have been the equivalent of a marathon or a 100-mile bike ride. All the sweat and tears along the way, all the hard work put in is well worth the reward. The moment you cross the finish line, it's as if all the energy spent running that marathon escapes your body and you collapse in exhaustion. The key to living a healthy lifestyle, you can't collapse. You have to keep going even after you reach your goal.

So, now that I have reached my 200-pound goal, what's next? That's easy. I am not through with my weight loss. Just like a marathon runner who finishes a marathon for the first time. They don't stop with just one marathon, especially if they are the type of person who wants to run in bigger marathons like the Boston or New York Marathons. Now

97

that I have lost my 200 pounds, I have decided it is time to reset my goal because now for me it is about reshaping my body composition, lowering my body fat percentage, getting off all of my prescription medications, especially insulin. My new weight loss goal is 30 pounds. Ultimately, I want to weigh 220 pounds.

For me to strive for that new goal, it will require me to think outside the box, which I have already started to do. I have started working out with a personal trainer, focusing more on strength training and not so much on cardio. You see, I have learned the last couple months that if you do strength training right, you can still have high-calorie burn while you are increasing your muscle mass. Thinking outside the box may also mean changing how I approach my nutrition, meaning adjusting my calorie intake so I am in a deficit which will help burn fat while increasing muscle mass. In doing so, I will continue losing weight and be able to maintain my weight loss long term. The idea of what I have been doing and continue to do is longevity of life. In other words, as long as the Lord gives me breath to breathe I want to have my health and wellness on point where I have the ability to be used by God to help other people reach their health and wellness goals, so they too can live a healthy lifestyle.

Thinking outside the box may also mean, doing things I wouldn't ordinarily do like flipping a tractor tire, leg pressing 240 pounds, pulling a weight sled 25 yards, or walking 3 minutes on a stair master. As I have been doing just this, I have noticed my calorie burn increasing when I do ride my bike. I can ride 20-25 miles and burn 1300 calories. I have also noticed small changes in my body composition. I'm starting to see muscle definition that I never imagined would be possible. I've noticed my arms and even my legs becoming more vascular, which that means I my circulation is improving, my blood is flowing better. This important because the pulmonary embolism, 13 years ago, really affected the circulation, especially in my left leg. My left calf muscle used to be much larger than my right calf muscle. While the left calf is still some bigger than the right, it isn't nearly as large as it used to be.

Early on in my journey it was about how many pounds, I was losing each week. The closer I get to the end of the journey it's been more about my body composition. Successful weight loss which is easy to sustain and maintain isn't just about the numbers. Understanding that lets me know that even if I go a week and only lose 1 pound or no weight at all, it's the other aspects I have to keep in mind. There should be no reason to get discouraged. It is important to surround yourself with people who will be there and pick you up when you fall. Then it becomes about responding to the adversity which comes along the way. Having the right pieces in place makes that much easier.

So, think out of the box when it comes to health and wellness. Change things up a bit after hitting a plateau. Change nutrition to match level of activity. Do less cardio and more strength training. It could mean putting yourself in a deficit, or it could mean increasing caloric intake with proper nutritional choices to help with muscle gain. If you look at it with this approach to avoid being stuck in a rut. Get out of that rut and think outside the box.

This isn't Just

The End

It's only the beginning

All you have to do is commit to the process and

dig roots, you will grow.

You can have all the passion in your heart but if

it's not clicking in your mind it doesn't matter, it

takes a change in mindset in order for the

journey to even begin.